Take Two Bones and Call Me In the Morning

Holistic First Aid for Dogs and Cats

Caroline O'Sullivan DVM, M.S.

First published by Dog Ear Publishing
4010 W. 86th Street, Ste H
Indianapolis, IN 46268
www.dogearpublishing.net

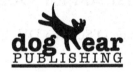

ISBN: 978-1-4575-3336-5

Library of Congress Control Number: has been applied for

This book is printed on acid-free paper.

Printed in the United States of America

Dedications

This book is dedicated to Michael James O'Sullivan Jr. Thank you for everything and I know you are here and guiding me and laughing the whole time. And to Gabriel and Hope, I truly wish I knew then what I know now. Thank you for motivating and teaching me.

Acknowledgments

I want to thank Alan for his kindness and patience. Thanks also to Ellen and Gary for editing, gentle constructive criticisms and their loving support.

Disclaimer

The information in this book is NOT intended to diagnose, treat, prevent or cure any medical conditions, nor is it intended to replace the personalized care of a licensed veterinarian.

CONTENTS

Part I – The Basics

Part II – Emergency Guide

Part III - References

PART I

The Basics

INTRODUCTION... My story

As I look back at the beginning of my journey as a veterinarian, I find that my work as a non-traditional practitioner started early with my student classification at Purdue Veterinary Medical School. As I was an older student, I was given the label "non-traditional" right away. Little did I know then that a terrible tragedy in my future would put me on the path to becoming "non-traditional" in everything I did.

Being accepted into veterinary medical school was difficult enough, but narrowing my focus was even harder, so, I decided that since I was there, I would do EVERYTHING. I jumped into a mixed rotation that included work with farm animals, equine, small animals (dog and cats), and I took every exotics course they offered. My externship in Tasmania allowed me access to many species of exotics as well as a look into how things were done outside the United States. Boy, did I learn!

After graduating from Purdue and passing the National Board Exam, I took a job in a small-animal practice in Las Vegas, and I performed the traditional Western medicine that I had learned in school. In the high-volume, twelve-doctor, on-call emergency hospital where I performed surgeries, gave vaccines, prescribed medications, and recommended diets, I believed completely in the care and advice I gave my patients and their caregivers.

One phone call changed everything, both professionally and personally.

My father, my Hero, was in the hospital, and it did not look good. He was a cardiovascular and thoracic surgeon, a commander of an aircraft carrier, a medical consultant and an attorney. If he was in the hospital, it was because he was performing surgery or seeing patients... until now.

This time, he was the patient. My dad had a dozen organ systems failing, a dozen separate specialists, with a dozen different treatment plans. My father was being treated as a list of problems, not as a whole man. In the end, nothing could save him and his death was slow and ugly.

For the six months of his hospitalization, I was traveling back and forth from Las Vegas to San Diego, trading the stresses of family, work and home. I continued to see veterinary patients during four 12-hour shifts at the clinic, took care of my own animals and home, and then drove to California.

After my father's death, I returned to my Western-style veterinary office and continued to treat my patients the way I always had. That is, until I overheard another doctor telling a pet parent, "I'm sorry, but there's nothing more I can do". All the frustration, helplessness, and anger that I had been carrying around with me came flooding out, and I said, "That's crap! There has to be something else we can do". I decided there and then that I was going to find it.

Immediately, I began to research, and I found the International Veterinary Acupuncture Society. From that moment on, I have been on a constant search for the "something else" that we as healers can use to help our patients, and every day since has been an adventure in education, information, and advocacy.

I truly believe that there is more out there that we can do. Where traditional, Western medicine is an integral part of solid medical care; there is a crucial place for holistic, nontraditional healing methods.

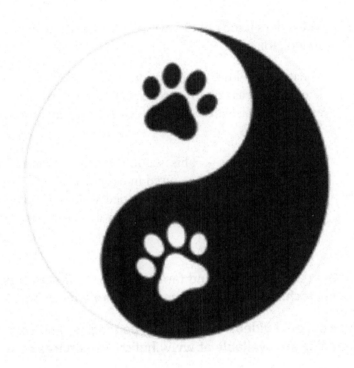

HOW TO USE THIS BOOK

This book is divided into chapters, each dealing with an emergency.

Each chapter has **four sections**:

1. What is it? Describes the specific issue / emergency.

2. What does it look like? Gives associated symptoms and what to look for.

3. What should I do? This section teaches techniques to stabilize your pet as you prepare to go to the veterinarian, if necessary. Here is where you will learn traditional thought and Western ideas.

4. Holistic Options - This section discusses non-traditional treatments that can be   used in conjunction with the traditional treatments, can be combined with traditional emergency procedures, and used on the way to the hospital.

⇨   **Please read this guide and familiarize yourself with these life-saving techniques BEFORE the time of an emergency.**

⇨   **Instructional videos on muzzling, bandaging, and controlling bleeding are available at www.holisticvetservices.com.**

Emergencies require immediate contact with your local veterinarian. Phone numbers should be posted in an easily accessible area and in cell phone directories.

When you call the vet, you'll need to describe the symptoms your pet is displaying, and be as specific as possible. Write down all advice and information given by the veterinarian and transport your pet to the hospital safely. First aid procedures may be started before and during transport to the hospital.

Tensions and emotions are running high during periods of emergencies for your loved ones. Having **the following supplies and information** at hand may help to make things go more smoothly:

1. Names, contact numbers, and locations of local emergency veterinary hospitals.

2. National Animal Poison Control Center phone number: 800-548-2423

   ASPCA Poison Control Center phone number: 888-426-4435

   Pet Poison Hotline: 888-681-3186

3. A portable first aid kit.

4. Phone numbers of friends and neighbors to assist in first aid and transport.

5. Attend First Aid and CPR classes offered in your area.

6. A soothing voice and some soft petting may help improve the emotional situation and give confidence to the patient.

7. Using acupressure: acupressure is the technique of applying direct pressure to specific locations (the meridians) on the body to achieve a desired effect. Pressure is applied for 30 - 90 seconds.

8. Homeopathy: operates from the premise of "treating like with like" – small, very diluted substances trigger the body's natural immune system to fight the symptoms that would manifest in a larger dose.

Acupressure is an integral part of this book – please note the proper way to place your finger for best results:

Acupressure – correct finger positioning
Drawn by Melissa Noor

| Correct | Incorrect | Incorrect |

Direct pressure should be applied to the skin with the finger held straight and firm. Do not apply too much pressure that might make your finger bend.

FIRST AID KIT

Be prepared ahead of time for any unforeseen accident with a good first aid kit, preferably a portable one that you can take with you anywhere.

The following are the basics of a first-rate, first aid kit:

1. Thermometer and lubrication - (normal dog and cat temperature is 101.5°, give or take a degree).

2. WaterRover - or other water container for easy access to hydration.

3. Coconut water - for natural sugars and electrolytes (restores Potassium, Magnesium, and Sodium).

4. Packet of Honey - restores blood sugar (good for hypoglycemia, collapse, shock, and dehydration).

5. Ginger tea - soothes upset stomach, vomiting and diarrhea. Cool before use.

6. Arnica 30C - for trauma and bruising.

7. Hypericum 30C - for superficial scrapes and nerve pain (back injuries and burns).

8. Belladonna 30C - helps decrease body temperature (poisonings and heat stroke).

9. Noni Lotion and Calendula - use as an antibacterial to promote wound healing.

10. Rescue Remedy - helps to decrease emotional and physical stress.

11. Alcohol pads - wipe over foot pads to bring down body temperature, wound   treatment.

12. Telfa pads - non-stick for wound wrapping.

13. Butterfly bandages.

14. Bandaging materials - gauze, Co-Flex, tape, cloth bandages.

15. Yunnan Bai Yao - (Hemostatic powder) to pour on bleeding wounds or to give   internally.

16. Eye Wash - Refresh eye drops, saline solution.

17. Blankets and Towels - for use in transport, to stop bleeding, and for warmth.

18. Pair of scissors and hemostats (tweezer-like clamps) - for removing stingers and splinters and to cut bandages.

19. Packets of granulated sugar and honey (unpasteurized) for wound care. Manuka honey is ideal.

⇨ **Complete First-Rate First Aid kits as well as Heatstroke kits are available for purchase at www.holisticvetservices.com. Containing all the essentials mentioned in this book's section on First Aid, they can help you keep your pet (or the pet of someone you care about) safe and healthy.**

MUZZLING

It is important to protect pets and humans from any injuries during times of emergencies, accidents, trauma, and transport. A leash or rope will help to make a soft muzzle, which will be used to make sure no bites occur as a result of fear or pain.

Signs of pain and anxiety vary among pets. Animals do not communicate signs of pain the way humans do, so we need to be aware of what to look for.

Some typical **signs of pain** are:

- Vocalizing

- Whining

- Going into hiding

- Trembling

- Agitation

- Restlessness

- Holding tail and head down

- Behavioral changes

- Snapping or biting when approached or touched

If you have any question about the comfort level or possible pain suffered by your pet, seek immediate veterinary attention, without getting hurt yourself.

⇨ **A soothing voice, reassuring words, acupressure points, and Rescue Remedy may help an uncomfortable or painful pet get to the hospital more easily.**

Muzzling

(Never muzzle an animal that is having difficulty breathing, is vomiting, or is unconscious. Using a blanket technique for transport can be more effective in these situations.)

1. While standing above and behind your pet, place a noose of material around the entire muzzle and pull the loop snug, but not tight. Your pet will need to be able to comfortably breathe and pant. (Muzzles can be made of gauze, a leash, a sock, a necktie, rope, a torn t-shirt, etc.).

2. Bring the edges of the material around behind the ears and tie in a bow.

3. Keep your hands away from the animal's mouth. To help relax your pet, gently stroke the area between its eyes starting near the nose and moving towards the ears. Your pet must be attended while muzzled, so it doesn't use its front paws to remove the muzzle. Always monitor for breathing comfort. If a pet has increased difficulty breathing while muzzled, the muzzle will need to be removed. Remember to keep your hand above and behind your pet's mouth.

Blanket Muzzling

If your dog is having difficulty breathing or is vomiting, a light towel or blanket can be used:

1. Standing behind and above your pet's head, slowly lower a lightweight towel, sheet or blanket over the pet's face. Apply no tension to the towel, but instead approach the pet from behind the ears and slip your hands around the neck and shoulder to make the patient feel relaxed and secure, with its mouth away from you.

2. Care must be taken with this technique, but the blanket can create a barrier to biting without restricting airflow as well as allowing the animal to vomit if needed.

Special Considerations for CATS

Cats require special handling considerations during an emergency, not only because they are smaller, but because they can be very quick at biting and scratching, especially when afraid or in pain.

1. Thick gloves should be used. The cat should be assessed for bleeding or for life-threatening wounds.

2. Towels can be used to wrap up the cat, with its legs safely inside the wrap.

3. The wrap can be secured with tape to prevent kicking and scratching, and to prevent further injuries.

4. Cats must be allowed to breathe with no obstruction to their noses (As cats are nose breathers, this is essential).

5. Cat muzzles are available, but they are sometimes difficult to apply.

Muzzling

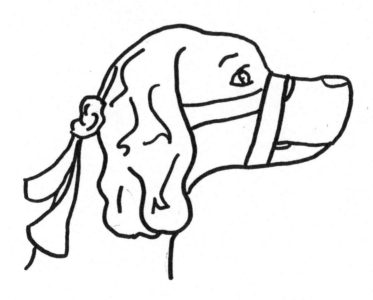

For a video on proper muzzling techniques, please visit www. youtube.com/user/DrODVM.

Wrapping Cat in a Towel

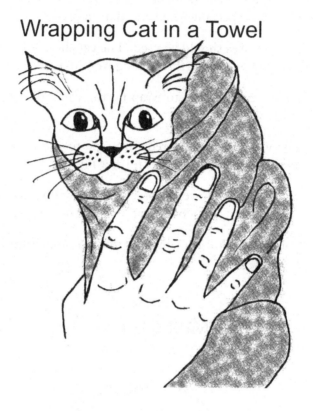

TRANSPORTATION OF INJURED PET

Flat boards

I n an effort to move your pet as little as possible during transportation, a firm, flat surface can be used to transport injured animals.

1. Pick a surface that will hold the pet's body weight.

2. Prepare to move the pet on this flat surface into a vehicle of appropriate size. Examples of a good flat surface include: a cutting board, plywood, an ironing board, a surfboard, etc. Transporting a 10lb cat is not the same as trying to move a 160 lb dog. Having access to an appropriate-sized vehicle is important. (I bought a Dodge Caravan with Stow-N-Go seating for my English Mastiffs after having an emergency situation. It is not the coolest vehicle on the road, but what a lifesaver!).

3. Place your pet gently on the board or slide the board under the pet.

   • Moving large animals can be difficult if they are unable to stand or are in crisis. I found that carefully sliding a sheet or blanket underneath them and then dragging them with the blanket onto the backboard or into the car makes a difficult task more manageable.

   • With smaller pets, a box or pet carrier may work nicely.

4. Gently secure your pet to the board. Sheets, clothing, towels, pillows, etc can all be used for this.

5. Having a friend to call is very important, it makes securing your pet for transport easier, provides emotional support for you and makes the drive much safer when one person is responsible for the pet and the other is responsible for the road.

6. Move your pet as little as possible, and try to move the entire pet as a unit. This means slow, smooth movements of the whole body into a secure location for transport.

CPR - The ABC's of Resuscitation

Always check for breathing and a pulse before starting CPR. Check pulses at inner thigh, below wrists and ankles, and over the heart. Check for breathing by looking for the chest to rise. Check the eyes. They may be dilated and the gums may be gray or white if the patient is not breathing and does not have a pulse.

Pulse Points

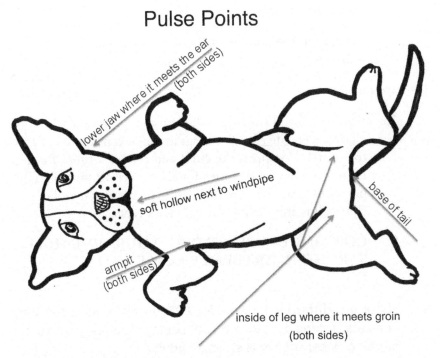

lower jaw where it meets the ear (both sides)

soft hollow next to windpipe

base of tail

armpit (both sides)

inside of leg where it meets groin (both sides)

"If there is no pulse, no breathing, no chest rise, and no movement, START the ABC's of CPR"

A – Airway

1. Lay your pet on a hard surface.

2. Extend the pet's neck forward, open its mouth and gently pull out the tongue.

3. Check the mouth and throat for any foreign material or vomit and carefully remove.

B - Breathing

4. Close the pet's mouth and gently hold it closed while blowing into the nostrils with 2 quick breaths until you see the chest rise. Use <u>only enough force</u> in breathing to get the chest to rise! If the breath goes in easily and makes the chest rise, continue to C-Circulation.

5. Release the mouth and nose and watch for the chest to fall. Continue to alternate between chest compression (Section C) and breathing.

6. Repeat until the pet breathes on its own or is given to a veterinarian.

C- Circulation

7. Place one hand over the other <u>on the chest wall where the elbow meets the ribs</u> (See diagram on next page) (location of the heart). Compress the chest and release 5 times for dogs up to 50 pounds, 10 times for dogs over 50 pounds (compressions must be less than 50% of the distance between your palms and the ground), THEN repeat step 4.

8. **CONTINUE CPR UNTIL YOUR PET HAS A STRONG HEARTBEART, PULSE AND IS BREATHING.**

⇨ **There are different models for CPR on different sized dogs and cats. Taking a   current CPR course through your veterinarian or local shelter is strongly advised.**

Muzzling instructions, transport techniques, and control of bleeding all may be needed during CPR.

Rescue Breathing

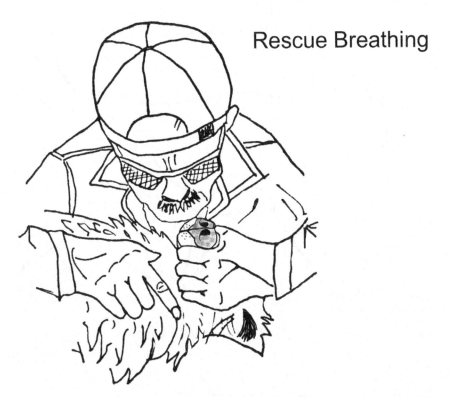

Gently hold your pet's mouth closed and breathe into its nose until you see the chest rise, then release.

CPR - Compression

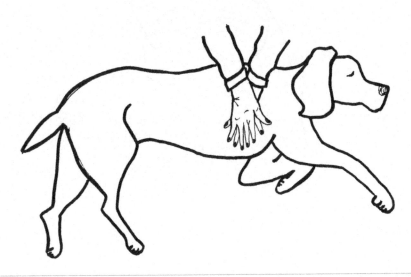

Cardiopulmonary Collapse

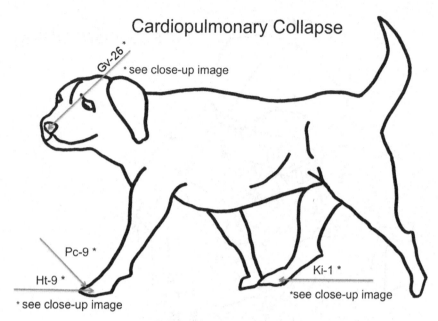

Gv-26 *
*see close-up image

Pc-9 *

Ht-9 *

Ki-1 *

*see close-up image

* see close-up image

5-30 minutes with CPR

Resuscitation Points

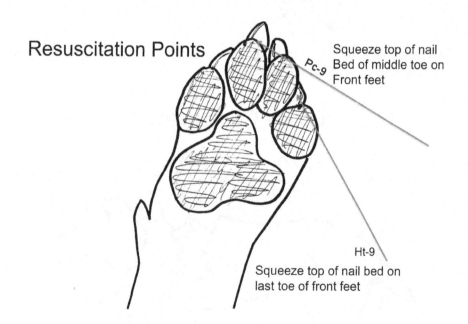

Pc-9

Squeeze top of nail
Bed of middle toe on
Front feet

Ht-9

Squeeze top of nail bed on
last toe of front feet

Resuscitation Point

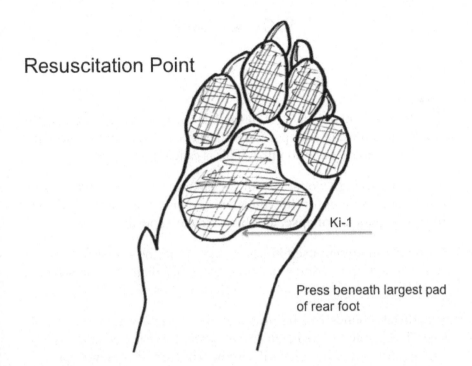

Ki-1

Press beneath largest pad
of rear foot

Resuscitation Point / "Hen Pecking"

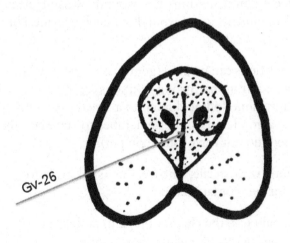

GV-26

Hen Pecking is rapid repeated jabs with a sharp object, like a pen or needle

WOUND CARE

During times of emergencies and unexpected events, assessing the situation and your pet as a whole is most important for deciding what gets medical attention first. This is called <u>triage</u>.

Sometimes seeing a wound on our pet can take the attention away from other more serious or life threatening concerns. **Always address bleeding, shock, collapse, and heat stroke-type signs first.**

A wound can present itself in many ways. It may be a superficial cut or scrape or a deep laceration or burn. Active bleeding and burns should be addressed as discussed in the chapters on those issues.

Superficial wounds can be protected and treated with a few simple steps. Deeper and more involved wounds will be handled at the veterinarian's discretion, but they will also benefit from these few steps:

- GENTLY rinse off wound with large amounts of water to remove dirt and debris - too much force in rinsing can drive debris and contaminants into the wound. Rinsing decreases bacterial contaminants in the wounds and will provide a healthy environment for healing.

- Antiseptic solutions can be used (gently) on superficial wounds, at diluted concentrations. <u>Strong solutions can actually damage tissue</u>. 1% Povidone Iodine diluted to a "weak-tea-color" concentration is a good antiseptic. Remember to rinse completely when finished (do not leave iodine on pet).

- Cover wounds with sterile, lint-free, nonstick pads to protect them from further contamination.

- Address the pain (see the chapter on pain) and discomfort, and try to keep your pet from licking the wound.

If a wound needs surgical closure, time is important. Ideally closure with debridement of the wound (the removal of dead or contaminated tissue) and sutures or staples should be performed in

the first 24 hours. After 48-72 hours, wound closures can become more complicated and healing time may be delayed.

If the wound cannot be closed or is a better candidate for healing without surgical intervention, it is called <u>Open Wound Management</u>, and it will require ongoing topical treatment, with possible bandaging and debridement by a veterinarian.

Holistic options:

- Arnica 30C will help with bruising, swelling, and discomfort. Can be given up to 3 times per day.

- Hypericum 30C will help address nerve pain of superficial wounds and grazing wounds. Give up to 3 times a day for stinging nerve pain.

- Noni Lotion – has proven antibiotic, antioxidant, and wound-healing properties. Can be applied directly to the wound and is safe if ingested orally.

- Aloe Vera – May accelerate wound healing and cooling skin

- Calendula Juice (diluted) or creams – May be antimicrobial and promote wound healing

Sweet Solutions:

Granulated Sugar can be used on wounds to reduce the bacterial load, help to remove necrotic (dead) tissue, absorb excess fluids from the wound, and promote healing.

- After wound is completely rinsed, a layer (1cm thick) of granulated sugar can be placed onto the wound and then be covered with a thick bandage. The sugar will draw fluids into the bandage materials.

- Bandage must be changed every 12-24 hours OR when fluid is visible on the outside of the bandage.

- Remove bandage, wound should be rinsed with large amounts of warm water or with saline.

- Re-apply granulated sugar and re-bandage. DO NOT LET PET EAT THE BANDAGE OR CONSUME LARGE AMOUNTS OF SUGAR.

- The fluids pulled from the wound may make your pet more prone to dehydration, so monitor drinking and keep large amount clean water available

Honey (unpasteurized) the hydrogen peroxide production and low pH promote wound healing.

- Soak a non-stick bandage in honey and apply to the wound, then apply another bandaging layer.

- Bandage must be changed daily and the wound cleaned with warm water and inspected before reapplication.

Allergic Reactions

Allergic reactions can have many different presentations. In this book, we will deal with three of the most common classifications of allergic reactions: stings and bites, food reactions, and vaccine reactions.

When animals are having an allergic reaction, they may present with one or more of the **following symptoms**:

- Hives

- Swelling

- Redness

- Itching

- Licking at a certain area

- Swelling around the eyes and face

- Vomiting

- Collapse

- Difficulty breathing

Stings and bites

When an animal has been bitten or stung, you need to:

1. Remove the stinger – Hemostats or tweezers are good for this task.

2. Apply an ice pack to the affected area for five minutes.

3. Proceed to an emergency hospital if you notice swelling around the head or face, hives, or difficulty breathing.

4. Benadryl can be given 1mg / pound twice daily (larger dogs start at ½ dose). Benadryl is safe for cats, although not very effective.

Holistic options:

- Ledum 6C every 30 minutes to address profound swelling.

- Apis 30C every hour until swelling subsides.

- Apple Cider Vinegar can be applied to area of inflammation, itch or sting. It is safe if pet licks apple cider vinegar.

- Place a fresh slice of onion on the area for quick relief. <u>Do NOT let your pet eat the onion or get it in the eye - it can cause blood and digestive disorders if ingested.</u>

Food reactions

Many allergic reactions to food result in vomiting and diarrhea. To help treat this, please refer to the sections on Vomiting and Diarrhea.

Holistic options:

- Withhold food for 12-24 hours.

- Continue small amounts of water, and add a teaspoon of coconut water for electrolytes.

- Nux Vomica 30C every 8-12 hours

- Urtica urens 30C for food allergy skin rashes

- Give room temperature ginger tea teaspoon-by-teaspoon to sooth the stomach.

- Acupressure points to relieve distress

Food Reactions

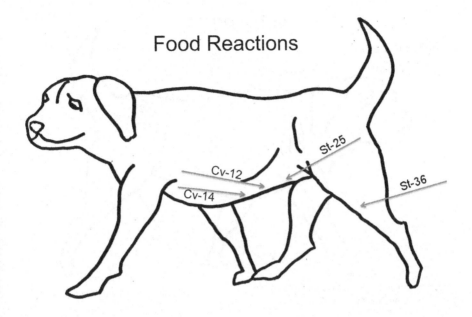

Cv-12
Cv-14
St-25
St-36

Diarrhea

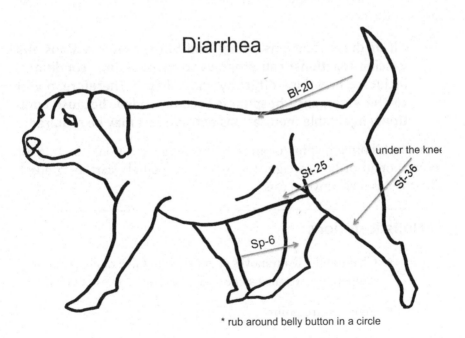

Bl-20
St-25 *
under the knee
St-36
Sp-6

* rub around belly button in a circle

Vomiting

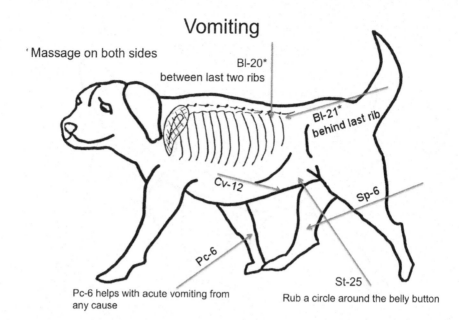

'Massage on both sides

Bl-20*
between last two ribs

Bl-21*
behind last rib

Cv-12

Sp-6

Pc-6

St-25

Pc-6 helps with acute vomiting from any cause

Rub a circle around the belly button

Vaccine reactions

A reaction to a vaccine usually presents as facial swelling, starting around the eyes.

⇨ **All of these reactions (stings and bites, food reactions and vaccine reactions) can progress to more serious conditions, including breathing difficulty and collapse, therefore, a visit to the emergency hospital is recommended, because additional injectable medications and support may be required.**

Benadryl is often helpful for any kind of allergic reaction. Use 1mg for every pound of body weight (dogs over 25 pounds start at ½ dose). Benadryl is ineffective in cats.

Holistic options:

- Chamomile Tea removes systemic itch. Give orally at room temperature. It can also be used topically in areas of itching.

- Acupressure points

- Ledum 6C every 30 minutes to address profound swelling

- Apis Mellifica 30C every hour until swelling subsides

BLEEDING

Loss of blood is a condition that requires **immediate attention**. It is important to know how to stop and/or slow the bleeding. Equally important is to know how to stop the bleeding WITHOUT CAUSING FURTHER HARM.

If you have a friend with you to help, have that friend apply a muzzle (as described in the chapter on muzzling), if appropriate, and call the emergency hospital.

Bleeding from a wound is normal. The majority of wounds will respond to a clean, dry pressure bandage. Bleeding should stop with direct pressure within five minutes.

Deep cuts may require sutures at the veterinarian's office.

Internal Bleeding

Some **signs of internal bleeding** may be extreme weakness, pale or white gums, distended abdomen, increased respiration, or blood coming from mouth, nose, urinary tract or anus. These patients may get cold and be thirsty. Body temperature under 100° is abnormal. The paws and ear tips may be cold.

- Yunnan Bai Yao - given orally will increase clotting inside the body (see page 32 for dosing information).

- Cover the pet with a blanket or towel to provide gentle warming.

- Get your pet to emergency veterinarian immediately.

External Bleeding

External Bleeding can come from many of the same causes in pets as it does in humans. There are three different types of bleeding:

1. **Superficial** – The bleeding stops by itself in 3-5 minutes. Your pet may lick the wound, which is okay as long as there

is no foreign body in the wound that your pet could swallow or cut its tongue on. These wounds can be gently rinsed with Betadine solution and a light wrap applied. **Clean and dry are the rules.**

2.   <u>Deep</u> - These wounds do not stop bleeding on their own within three minutes and may produce a large volume of blood. This requires a pressure bandage (to slow and stop the bleeding. Yunnan Bai Yao may also be applied to the wound before applying pressure. <u>The pressure bandage should be kept in place for short periods of time and checked often to avoid loss of circulation</u>. See below for instructions on how to apply a pressure bandage.

3.   <u>Artery or venous bleeding</u> – if a major blood vessel is cut, direct pressure on the wound and pressure bandages may not be enough. A tourniquet may need to be placed between the body and the wound to slow the blood leaving the blood vessel. THIS CONDITION REQUIRES AN EMERGENCY ROOM. Call the emergency animal hospital and tell them you are coming in order to save time and get their advice for transportation.

The **following techniques** are to be used in order, for five minutes, before moving onto the next technique:

1.   Apply direct pressure to the bleeding area. Raise the area that is bleeding above the level of the heart, if possible. How to apply a **pressure bandage**:

   • Place a piece of clean cloth over the area that's bleeding and apply flat pressure with your hands. If needed, place a second cloth, without disturbing the first cloth, and continue the steady pressure on the wound.

   • When the bleeding stops, apply a clean, soft bandage.

   • If a second cloth continues to seep, gently wrap vet wrap or an Ace bandage around the injury to secure the compress over the bleeding wound. DO NOT CUT OFF CIRCULATION COMPLETELY.

2.   IF THE BLEEDING DOESN'T STOP, see if the blood is spurting out (arterial bleeding) or if there is a steady heavy

flow (venous bleeding). Apply a secure compress tightly over the bleeding wound, then:

- With spurting blood (arterial bleeding), apply pressure to the pet's pressure points that lie <u>between</u> the wound and the animal's body, while continuing direct pressure on the wound (see illustration below).

- With heavy flow without spurting (venous bleeding), apply pressure to the pet's pressure points that lie <u>below</u> the wound (away from the body) while continuing direct pressure on the wound.

⇨ **Pressure points** are the points on the body where blood vessels originate.

3. <u>Tourniquets</u> **(use only as last resort after the other techniques have been tried.)** A tourniquet can cause damage to the area on which it is being used. ONLY USE ON LIMBS AND TAILS.

Pressure from a tourniquet needs to be loosened for 10-20 seconds every 2-3 minutes. This allows **critical blood to flow** to the area below the tourniquet.

- Place a wide piece of cloth or gauze around the area above the bleeding wound. Wrap it around twice.

- Take the loose ends of the material and wrap it around a rigid object (tongue depressor, stick, pencil, etc) and twist the rigid object slowly and watch for the bleeding to stop. Do not twist any further than needed.

Holistic options:

- Arnica and Phosphorus 30C work well for hemorrhage.

- Calendula, aloe and Noni Lotion can be applied to *superficial cuts* and may help slow bleeding and bacteria growth, aid in skin comfort and promote healing.

- Arnica 30C can be used to slow bruising and swelling while promoting healing. Hypericum 30C is helpful in cases of skin grazes and superficial wounds.

- Yunnan Bai Yao can be used during and after any bleeding crisis. Yunnan Bai Yao can be applied directly to wounds to stop bleeding and form a clot. <u>Oral doses for internal bleeding cases</u>: (Dogs) less than 30 lbs – 1 capsule twice a day. Dogs 30-60 lbs – 2 capsules twice a day. Dogs over 60 lbs – 2 capsules three times a day. Cats ½ capsule twice a day.

- It can be used during and after any bleeding crisis, both internally and topically.

- Arnica 30C can be given every 4 hours for one day to decrease soft tissue shock and promote healing.

- Aconitum for sudden hemorrhage.

- Acupressure points for stress

Pressure Points

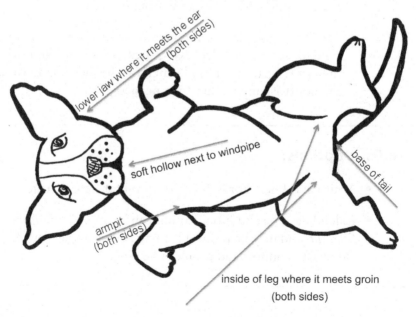

lower jaw where it meets the ear (both sides)

soft hollow next to windpipe

base of tail

armpit (both sides)

inside of leg where it meets groin (both sides)

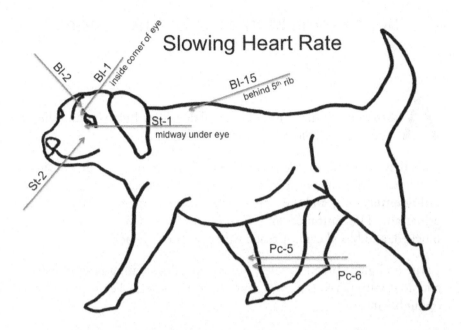

Slowing Heart Rate

Bl-2

Bl-1

inside corner of eye

Bl-15
behind 5th rib

St-1
midway under eye

St-2

Pc-5

Pc-6

These points aid in relaxation during times of stress:

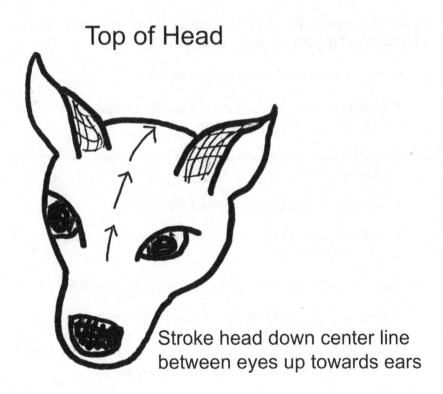

Top of Head

Stroke head down center line
between eyes up towards ears

BLOAT – The Mother of All Emergencies

A distended stomach full of gas will develop a bulge behind the rib cage causing "bloat" or Gastric Dilation.

This may result in the bloated stomach twisting upon itself, causing a "volvulus" (stomach twisting upon itself). The volvulus is a **life-threatening emergency** and the **only option** is an emergency trip to the veterinarian. The entrance and exit of the stomach are twisted and blocked, and blood cannot reach other parts of the body.

Large and giant breeds, males, older dogs, dogs with a family history, and dogs with nervous personalities have an increased chance of developing bloat.

All dogs, and even cats, can bloat - please read this section multiple times to be prepared!

TIME IS LIMITED AND SURGERY MAY BE THE ONLY THING TO HELP YOUR PET SURVIVE!

The following are **typical symptoms** to look for:

- Non-productive retching is the number one sign. A dog will try to vomit and nothing comes up.

- Restlessness, pacing, unable to get comfortable, panting, digging holes.

- Swelling of the abdomen behind the rib cage.

- If the stomach twists, there will be extreme pain and collapse and probable death.

While you are making plans to go to the emergency hospital:

- Simethicone (found in Gax-X) can help reduce the stomach swelling before the "volvulus" occurs, or possibly keep it from becoming more bloated with gas. Do this **IMMEDIATELY** when you notice any of the above symptoms.

- <u>Doses for dogs</u>: Small dogs: ¼ human dose, medium dogs ½ human dose, large dogs 1-2 pills

- Call your local emergency veterinarian and describe the symptoms and let them know that you are on your way.

  Call a friend to help transport your pet.

Holistic options:

- Lycopodium 30c is helpful with gassy bloated stomach

- Single dose Alumina 30 then Carbo Vegetabilis 30C every 15 minutes on the way to the Emergency Vet

- Nux Vomica 30C every 15 minutes until risk of torsion has passed.

- Acupressure Stomach Points

Stomach Points

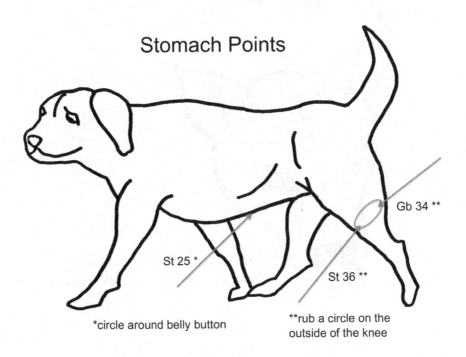

Gb 34 **

St 25 *

St 36 **

*circle around belly button

**rub a circle on the outside of the knee

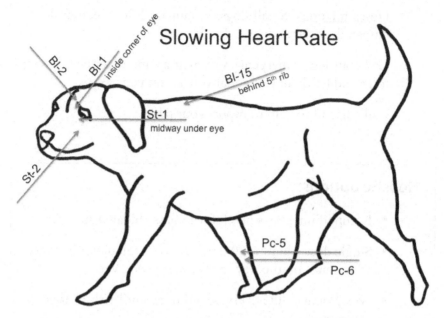

Slowing Heart Rate

Acupressure points that are good for calming your pet during transport:

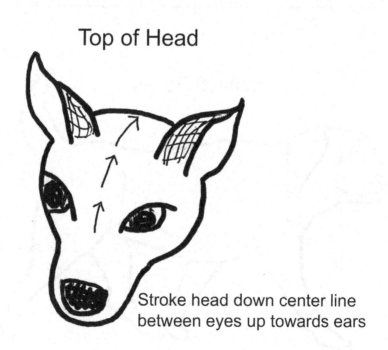

Top of Head

Stroke head down center line between eyes up towards ears

BROKEN BONES AND DISLOCATIONS

This requires the care of skilled veterinarians. DO NOT TRY TO RESET THE BONE!

Broken Bones and dislocations

Severe pain can be expected with a fracture or dislocation of any kind. Applying a muzzle and gently restraining your pet are the first things needed. Pain control, a stretcher, or a splint will be needed to transport your pet for further care at a veterinary hospital. NEVER try to reposition the limb. **The goal is to decrease movement from the current position.**

1. Create a splint by wrapping the limb in loose material (such as cotton), then in a thick roll of cotton, clothes, newspaper, a magazine, etc., and finally taping the thick roll into place.

2. **The splint must extend one joint <u>above</u> and one joint <u>below</u> the area of fracture or dislocation. Restraining your pet in a carrier or on a flat surface is best, if your pet will remain quiet and still in the carrier or flat surface.**

3. If the animal is moving a lot, place a towel between the skin and the newspaper splint to keep from forming a skin sore.

Holistic options:

- While waiting to receive veterinary care, Arnica 30C can be used orally immediately and every 2 - 4 hours thereafter to reduce the risk of shock.

- After a licensed veterinarian has addressed the bones, Symphyum 1x can be used 1 – 3 times after the injury for one week, then once daily for the next few weeks at 12C to promote healing.

- For injuries involving nerves, Hypericum 30C every 8 -12 hours is most helpful.

- Rescue Remedy can be given for stress. Place a couple drops on nose, gums and temple.

Open fractures

An open fracture has resulted when a bone has protruded from the skin. If this has occurred, soak gauze or a clean cloth in saline solution or water. Apply the soaked cloth or gauze gently to the area and tape it in place before securing the splint.

Broken tails

1. Stop the bleeding (see the chapter on Bleeding).

2. Wash wounds with mild soap and warm water.

3. Apply a non-stick sterile gauze pad.

4. Wrap the tail from tip to base with first aid tape or cohesive flexible bandage, including a rigid object (stick, utensil, chop stick, etc.) inside the tail wrap. Be careful not to cut off circulation while wrapping tail gently.

5. Your veterinarian will determine treatment depending upon break locations and long-term effects (tail base fractures sometimes lead to permanent difficulty in lifting the tail, nerve damage, difficulty in wagging the tail and decreased feeling).

Materials to keep in a kit for stabilizing broken bones:

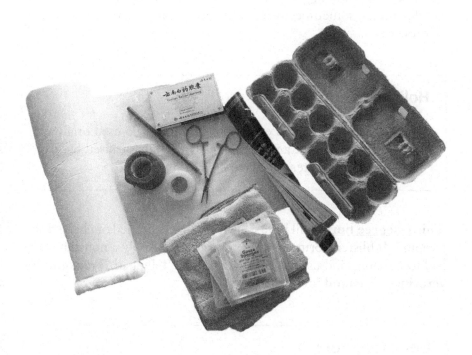

Gauze, tape, scissors, Yunnan Bai Yao, cotton cloths, rigid stick (for splint), egg crate, magazine, newspaper, etc. (to wrap around the limb).

BURNS

There are three kinds of burns: heat burns, chemical burns and electrical burns.

Heat, chemicals and electricity can cause first, second, and third-degree burns. These are all painful conditions and need to be treated immediately.

First and second-degree burns will be red, may be painful to the touch, and are sometimes swollen. At-home care can usually take care of these cases.

Holistic option:

- Urtica urens 30C every four hours can be used orally or dilute in water and use topically on burns caused by fire, heat, and water scalds.

Third-degree burns will have white skin that is burned or charred and weeping. If blisters form, do not rupture them. Apply a nonstick Telfa pad to the area, and use an ice pack over the Telfa pad. **Transport to veterinary hospital immediately.**

Holistic option:

- Cantharis 6C may be a helpful homeopathic for blisters.

Heat burns - (usually from water or oil) Place the burned area under *low-pressure*, cold running water. Too much water pressure can damage the already-damaged skin. Ice packs can also be used for 2 minutes on, 3 minutes off intervals. These treatments should last 20 minutes. Apply ointment and dress the wound.

Chemical burns - (usually from household and yard products) – Flood the area with lots of water to dilute the chemical. Continue to flood and dilute the area even if the skin starts to change in color or texture.

Transport the animal to a hospital. Acupressure points for relaxation may help during transport.

You can call the poison hotlines for help with chemical burns. (Phone numbers are in the front of this book).

Electrical burns - (usually happens when a pet bites into an electrical cord) – depending on the amount of electrical charge and the time of exposure, the pet may show symptoms ranging from a bad taste in its mouth to lung damage, with coughing, drooling, and difficulty breathing, or even respiratory arrest.

In the case of respiratory arrest, begin CPR and arrange for immediate transport to the hospital (see the section on CPR at the front of this book).

Symptoms may be delayed for days. Watch for reluctance to eat, drooling, bad smell from the mouth, anxiety, and tissues in the mouth flaking off.

Holistic options:

- Aloe, Noni Lotion, and Calendula are safe, soothing topicals for burns.

- Acupressure

- Slippery elm tea with Arnica 30C makes a nice oral flush

Burns

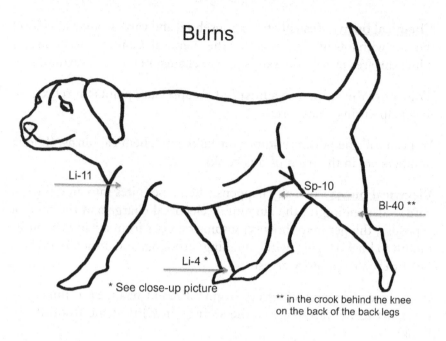

Li-11

Sp-10

BI-40 **

Li-4 *

* See close-up picture

** in the crook behind the knee
on the back of the back legs

Li-4

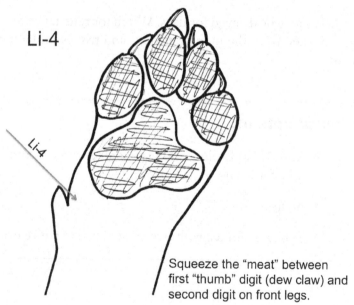

Li-4

Squeeze the "meat" between
first "thumb" digit (dew claw) and
second digit on front legs.

These points help release heat in the body.

CHOKING

W hen your pet swallows a toy or a big piece of food or bone, they choke the same way that humans do, so we use the same treatments.

If an animal is choking, you may notice that it is having difficulty breathing and is coughing, gagging, and becoming agitated and anxious while rubbing at its face to try to dislodge the item.

Use the **following techniques** to assist your pet:

1. Lift the pet's rear end off the ground gently, like a wheelbarrow, and shake. If the pet is small enough, it can be lifted completely off the ground with its head down.

2. Heimlich – With the animal's back against you, wrap your arms around the belly right beneath the ribs and give one forceful squeeze (in and up).

3. Remove the object - without oxygen, the pet may faint. If this happens, open its mouth, extend the neck, pull the tongue forward, and remove the object.

4. If you are unable to remove the object, go straight to the emergency veterinarian.

5. Perform CPR if the pet stops breathing and has no pulse (see the section on CPR at the front of this book).

Holistic options:

- Aconitum can be given after a choking incident.

Choking

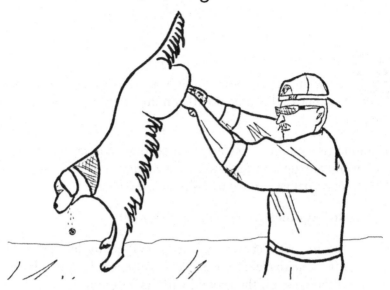

Heimlich Maneuver

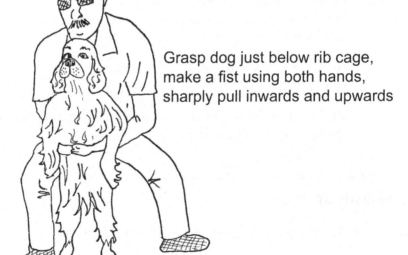

Grasp dog just below rib cage, make a fist using both hands, sharply pull inwards and upwards

DIARRHEA

Stool that has any abnormal consistency, odor, mucous coating, or blood is abnormal. Pets can lose large amounts of body water if diarrhea persists, which can be a secondary serious challenge to your pet's health and ability to recovery.

If your pet's diarrhea continues for more than 12 hours, or if your pet becomes tired, disoriented, or weak, <u>seek veterinary assistance immediately</u>. Always see a veterinarian if there is blood present in the stool.

There are some **common symptoms** that can indicate the presence of diarrhea in your pet:

- Abdominal pain
- Loud stomach sounds
- Food in the stool
- Little to no appetite
- Foul-smelling stool
- Mucous or blood on the stool
- Flatulence
- Straining to defecate

Some **signs of dehydration** can be:

- Dry gums
- Low desire to drink
- Dark urine in small quantity
- Coughing

<u>If you suspect dehydration, contact the veterinarian immediately</u>.

When your pet is suffering from diarrhea, **you should**:

- Maintain hydration with water and electrolytes, using coconut water or electrolyte drinks in small amounts.

- Bring a fecal sample to your vet to check for intestinal parasites.

- Add bulk to your pet's diet with insoluble fibers such as pumpkin, although not pumpkin pie filling due to its high sugar content.

- Begin probiotics that are labeled for use in dogs and cats.

Holistic options:

- Glutamine helps support the health of the gastrointestinal tract.

- Slippery Elm with probiotics works well for cats and dogs (1/4 teaspoon per 10 pounds twice per day).

- Decrease the diet to one simple protein and one simple carbohydrate (i.e. chicken and rice) in small amounts multiple times per day.

- Kudzu root

- Marshmallow Root and Leaves can help diarrhea with straining, blood, and mucous.

Diarrhea

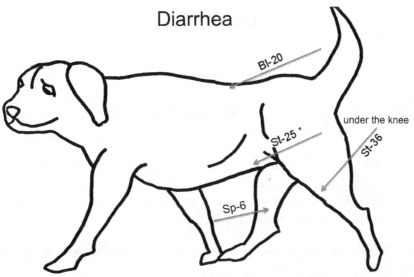

BI-20

under the knee

St-25 *

St-36

Sp-6

* rub around belly button in a circle

DROWNING

Your pets should always be **monitored around water**, no matter how proficient they are at swimming or are "water dogs" by breed.

A small dog falling into a pool with high edges, a dog swimming too far out in a lake or ocean to make it back to shore without exhaustion, or a pet falling through the ice are just some of the countless ways drowning can claim the life of your beloved friend.

The **following techniques** will help your pet in a drowning situation:

1. If you find your pet in the water and unconscious, pull him out and gently swing him by his back legs with his head down to drain the water from the lungs. This should allow breathing to begin.

2. With larger dogs, you may need to keep the front feet on the ground (like a wheelbarrow) and raise the back legs and shake to remove water from the lungs.

3. Next place the pet on the ground on its side with a cushion under the hind end so that the head is lower than the body, clear the mouth, and tilt the head back to open the airway.

4. If the pet is not breathing, and has no pulse, begin CPR (see the section on CPR at the front of this book).

5. Take the pet to the veterinarian. Even if the pet is resuscitated, treatments may be needed to prevent pneumonia.

Dogs that go swimming or are riding in a boat should always wear a life vest.

Holistic options:

- Aconitum is helpful to give following a drowning incident.

- Phosphorous 30C - 1 pellet every 4 hours. Good for addressing inflammation of the respiratory tract.

Drowning

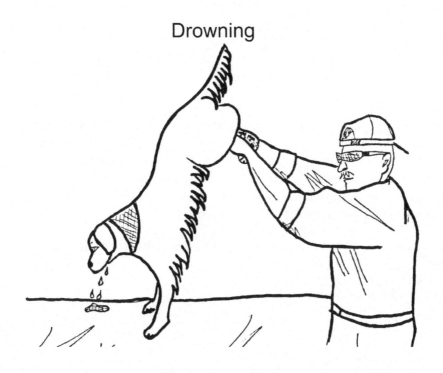

Looking snazzy and safe in his life vest

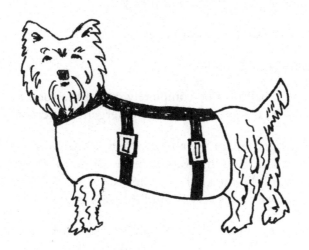

EYE INJURIES

njuries to the eye can happen anytime, from the wind blowing material into the eye, a scratch from a stick or another pet, glaucoma, an aggressive rub of the paw on the head, or from blunt-force trauma. Some animals are more prone to eye injuries because the globes of their eye protrude more than other animals. Pugs and Chihuahuas are good examples of dogs that have eyes that protrude.

When an animal has injured its eye, there are **indicators** you can look for:

- Blinking rapidly

- Holding the eyes shut

- Excessive tearing

- Rubbing at the eyes

- Redness in the white part of the eye

- Inability to shut eye completely

- Possibly crying and lethargy

Sometime the eyeball may be completely out of the socket. THIS IS AN EMERGENCY! Go directly to the emergency veterinarian.

- If you notice any of the above symptoms, you can gently flush the eye with running water, sterile saline or human contact solution (NOT the kind with the red tip – this is used for protein removal and is very painful if it gets in the eye).

- Keep the eye moist with KY Jelly, sterile saline solution or wet compresses ONLY. Other solutions could hurt the eye tissue.

- **Get to the veterinary hospital as soon as possible**, because the eyesight of your pet is extremely valuable. Eye injuries worsen rapidly!

Holistic options:

- Mercurius corrosivus for scrapes or scratches on the cornea.

- Ledum is helpful when the entire eye is injured.

- Arnica 30C for pain and swelling.

- Euphrasia 30C for pain and cloudy eyes.

- Acupressure

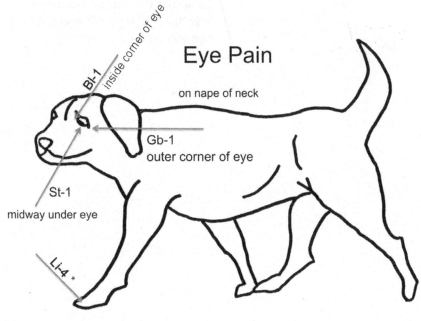

Eye Pain

Bl-1
inside corner of eye

on nape of neck

Gb-1
outer corner of eye

St-1
midway under eye

Li-4 *

*see close-up image

Li-4

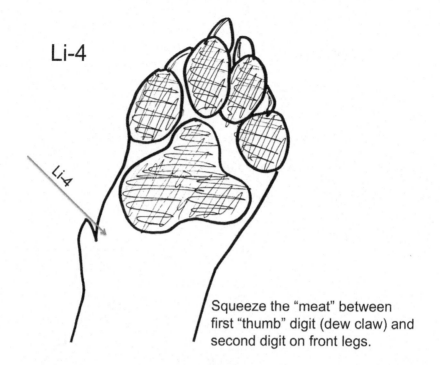

Squeeze the "meat" between first "thumb" digit (dew claw) and second digit on front legs.

HEATSTROKE

NEVER LEAVE YOUR PET IN A CAR IN THE SPRING, SUMMER, OR FALL.

A closed car can reach 120° F. Animals only cool down by panting and do not sweat to get rid of heat. Brain damage and internal organ dysfunctions begin when the body gets to 106° F.

Dogs can suffer from a walk on a hot day or in a yard with no shade, especially if they have any respiratory problems or they have a short muzzle.

Signs of heat stroke include:

- Frantic panting

- Anxiety

- Red tongue

- Thick saliva

- Glazed eyes

- Warm foot pads

- Vomiting

- Diarrhea

- Dizziness

- High body temperature

Animals suffering from heat stroke must be **cooled down,** but not too rapidly.

1.   Drape your pet with a wet towel.

2.   Use a digital thermometer to check temperature (anything over 102.5° F is abnormal).

3. Use a hose to wet the pet down for 1-2 minutes.

4. Get the pet into an air-conditioned room.

5. Offer cold water.

6. Spray rubbing alcohol on the pads of the feet.

7. Call the emergency vet and describe your pet's symptoms.

8. Rub ice on your pet's gums and on its feet. Be cautious around the mouth, as the animal may bite from distress.

9. Point a fan in the pet's direction.

10. Transport your pet to a hospital for evaluation. THIS IS ESSENTIAL.

Holistic options:

- Aconite 30C for signs of acute heatstroke including restlessness, agitation and fearful behaviors.

- Glonoinium if the animal seems listless or in a stupor.

- Belladonna 6C if eyes are glazed and pupils dilated. Every 2 hours.

- Use Rescue Remedy around mouth and gums to reduce stress.

- Herbal calming sprays - spray in the environment, not on your pet.

- Pressure points - Acupuncture (heat releasing points).

⇨   **Heatstroke kits are available at www.holisticpetservices.com.**

Heatstroke

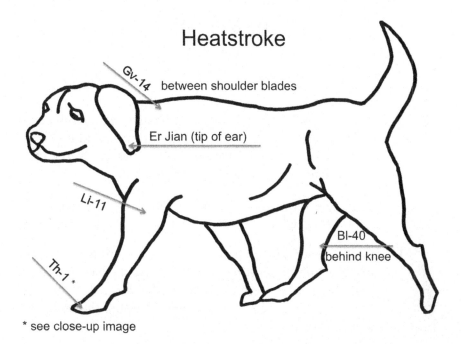

Gv-14 between shoulder blades

Er Jian (tip of ear)

LI-11

BI-40 behind knee

Th-1 *

* see close-up image

Th-1

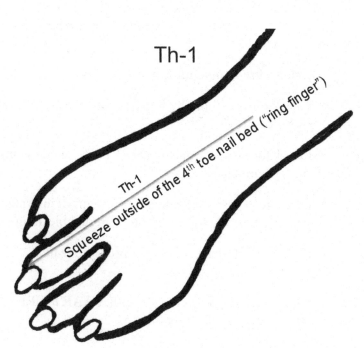

Th-1 Squeeze outside of the 4th toe nail bed ("ring finger")

clears heat from the body

HIT BY CARS

U nfortunately, this type of emergency happens all too often. The trauma suffered by the animal can be obvious, internal, and delayed. Often, there are skin and soft-tissue injuries, broken or dislocated bones, internal injuries, bleeding, and shock.

Assume that these victims are scared and in pain. They may want to run away or lash out. Proceed with caution, compassion, and extreme care.

1. Get your pet out of the street. Remember to move the animal as a unit by scruffing the hair along the back (one hand grab the scruff of neck and the other grab the skin above the hips) and dragging it out of danger, keeping the body even with the road.

2. Muzzle the pet if possible, for both your and your pet's protection (see section on muzzling at the beginning of this book).

3. Check for breathing, pulse, and bleeding.

   • Check for breathing by watching for rise and fall of chest or for panting.

   • Check for pulse by placing your hand high on the inside of the back limbs.

   • Check for external bleeding, or for signs of internal bleeding (see chapter on bleeding for internal bleeding signs).

   • If there is bleeding, follow the procedures in the bleeding chapter.

IF THERE IS NO BREATHING OR PULSE, **START CPR** (see the section on CPR at the front of this book).

4. Keep the pet covered and warm.

5. Stabilize any broken or dislocated bones (see chapter on broken bones and dislocations)

6. Get your pet to an emergency veterinarian.

7. Buffered aspirin can be used for short-term relief of pain or inflammation. **Never use in cats**. Give every 12 hours. Aspirin can cause thinning of the blood.

Holistic option:

- Use Rescue Remedy on temple, nose, and gums to help reduce panic, shock, and emotional stress.

- Aconite 30C plus Arnica 30C

- Star of Bethlehem flower to reduce shock and stress.

- Acupressure for pain and shock

Pain

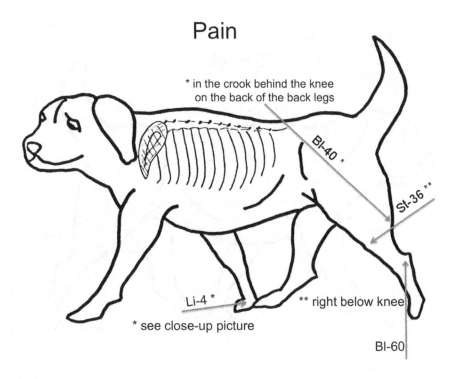

* in the crook behind the knee on the back of the back legs

Bl-40 *

St-36 **

Li-4 *

** right below knee

* see close-up picture

Bl-60

Li-4

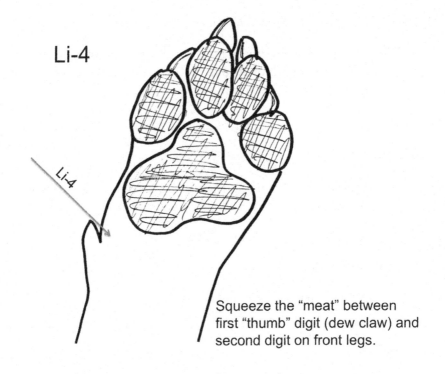

Squeeze the "meat" between first "thumb" digit (dew claw) and second digit on front legs.

Shock

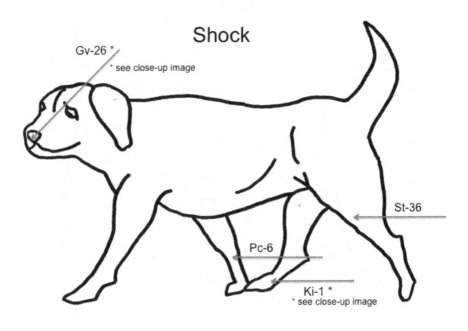

Gv-26 *
* see close-up image

St-36

Pc-6

Ki-1 *
* see close-up image

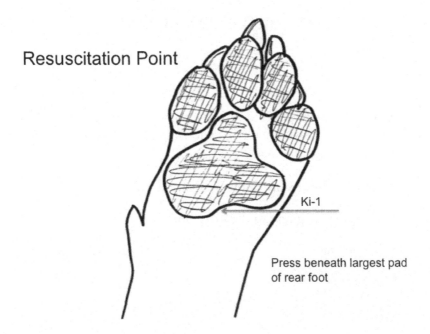

Resuscitation Point

Ki-1

Press beneath largest pad
of rear foot

Resuscitation Point / "Hen Pecking"

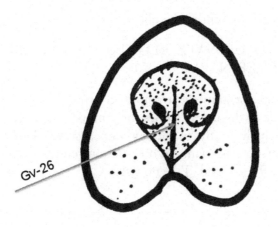

GV-26

Hen Pecking is rapid repeated jabs with a sharp object, like a pen or
needle

INABILITY TO URINATE

nability to urinate can be a serious problem for both cats and dogs. Cats that have this difficulty can actually be obstructed, which is a very painful and life-threatening situation.

You may notice **these symptoms** in your animal:

- Cats may be going to the litter box repeatedly.

- Vocalizing

- Vomiting

- Showing agitation

- Straining to urinate, with little or no results

- Blood in the urine

- Cats may be licking under the tail

AN INABILITY TO URINATE REQUIRES AN IMMEDIATE TRIP TO THE VETERINARIAN.

Other reasons for animals straining to urinate may be infections, crystals in the urine, stones, or tumors. The only way to determine which, if any, of these is the cause will be through testing at the veterinarian. An obstruction requires veterinary intervention for survival. Take no risks.

Holistic options:

- Saw Palmetto (extract, not powder) can be used to ease spasms of the urethra, increase comfortable urine flow, and helps reduce obstructions. Give 1cc every 30 min until cat urinates. Then continue at 1-2 ml twice a day until problem is resolved.

- Aconitum for painful difficulties with urination and issues with a sudden onset.

- Cantharis 30C for blood in the urine and pain associated with problems urinating.

- Hydrangea 30C can aid in breaking up deposits, especially in cats. Give every 30 min until cat urinates.

- Acupressure is very helpful in cases of cats straining to urinate.

Inability to Urinate

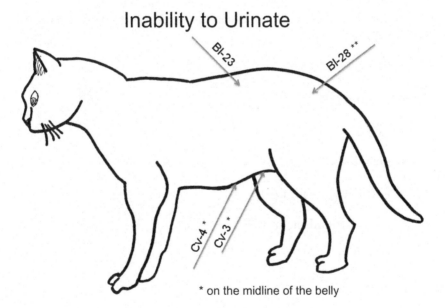

* on the midline of the belly

POISONING

Pets have a habit of getting into all kinds of items that are no good for them.

The phrase "dog proofing" or "pet proofing" your house is sometimes easier said than done. Even if you use childproof devices on drawers, cabinets, garage shelving, and bathroom doors, your dog will still find little things to eat that can lead to big problems.

Your pet doesn't always have to eat the poison for it to affect him. Poisons that find their way onto the animal's feet or coat may be ingested during grooming or licking, or they can simply penetrate the skin.

Even if you do not see your pet eat a poison, here are **some symptoms** that you should watch out for:

- Seizures

- Bleeding

- Vomiting/Diarrhea

- Drooling

- Difficulty breathing

- Burns around the mouth

- Staggering

- Foaming at the mouth

<u>Time is of the utmost importance when our pets have been exposed to poisons.</u>

Immediately.....

1. Identify the substance your pet consumed.

2. Call the **ASPCA Poison Control at 888-426-4435** or the **National Animal Poison Control Center at 800-548-**

2423. They are open 365 days a year, 24 hours a day. They will give you instructions on how to care for your pet and give you a case number.

3. Call your emergency vet, tell them what has happened and give them the case number you just received. This allows your veterinarian to get all the necessary information from poison control, and the hospital can be getting ready for the treatment of your pet while you are en route.

4. Inducing vomiting is the best way to get the substance out of your pet's system, BUT MANY SUBSTANCES WILL CAUSE MORE DAMAGE COMING BACK UP IN THE VOMIT.

    • The substance consumed must be identified <u>before</u> the decision to induce vomiting is made.

    • Time of consumption and exposure are important as well. If time has passed, an antidote used to dilute the poison or decrease its absorption may be best.

    • <u>Always</u> consult Poison Control or your veterinarian before inducing vomiting.

    • To induce vomiting: use a 3% solution of Hydrogen Peroxide at a dose of 1 teaspoon per ten pounds of body weight every 20 minutes. Use twice and then call for further instructions.

5. Bring the container that held the poison to the veterinarian or have it ready to discuss with Poison Control.

6. Bleeding should be addressed with pressure and Yunnan Bai Yao (see the chapter on bleeding for more information).

7. Any burns on the body should be address as described in the chapter on burns.

Holistic options:

- Homeopathic Remedies such as Nux Vomica 30C and Arsenicum 30C can be considered after the emergency is over to help eliminate toxins and support the digestive system.

- Acupressure can be used for nausea, vomiting, diarrhea, collapse, and seizures.

Vomiting

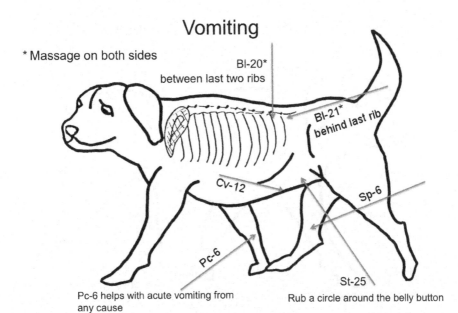

* Massage on both sides

Bl-20*
between last two ribs

Bl-21*
behind last rib

Cv-12

Sp-6

Pc-6

St-25

Pc-6 helps with acute vomiting from any cause

Rub a circle around the belly button

Diarrhea

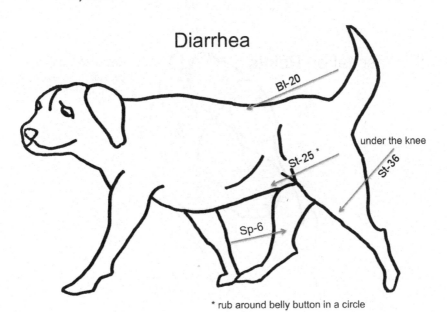

Bl-20

under the knee

St-25 *

St-36

Sp-6

* rub around belly button in a circle

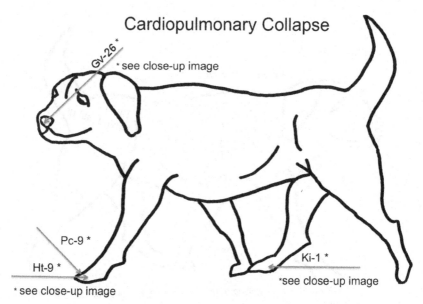

Cardiopulmonary Collapse

Gv-26 *
* see close-up image

Pc-9 *

Ht-9 *
* see close-up image

Ki-1 *
*see close-up image

5-30 minutes with CPR

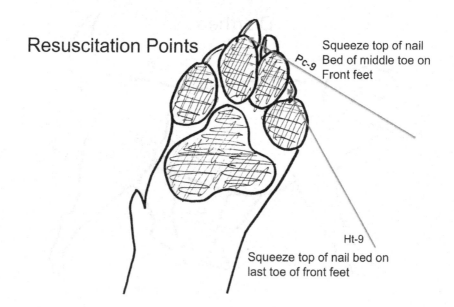

Resuscitation Points

Pc-9
Squeeze top of nail
Bed of middle toe on
Front feet

Ht-9
Squeeze top of nail bed on
last toe of front feet

Resuscitation Point

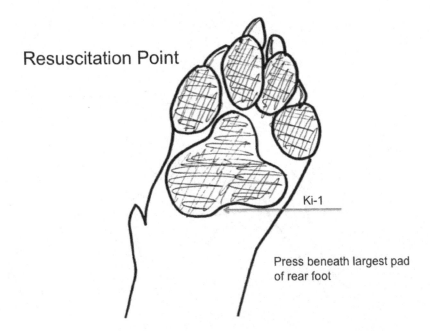

Ki-1

Press beneath largest pad
of rear foot

Resuscitation Point / "Hen Pecking"

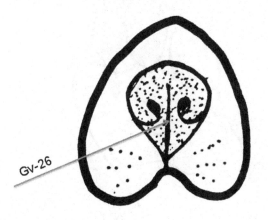

Gv-26

Hen Pecking is rapid repeated jabs with a sharp object, like a pen or needle

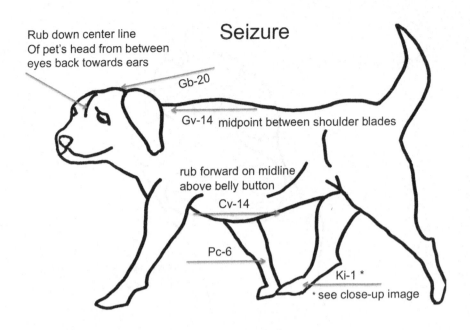

Seizure

Rub down center line
Of pet's head from between
eyes back towards ears

Gb-20

Gv-14 midpoint between shoulder blades

rub forward on midline
above belly button

Cv-14

Pc-6

Ki-1 *

* see close-up image

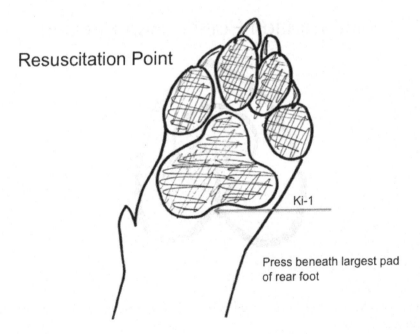

Resuscitation Point

Ki-1

Press beneath largest pad
of rear foot

Top of Head

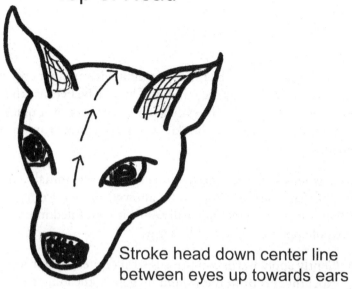

Stroke head down center line between eyes up towards ears

PUNCTURE WOUNDS

These wounds can be the result of a fight with another creature and may be difficult to locate initially. This can be because the wound may just be a small break in the skin, and it may cover over quickly, hiding the damaged areas where the skin was moved away from the underlying tissues.

Puncture wounds become easily infected by the initial injury and require draining, cleaning, and to be allowed to heal <u>from the inside out</u>. Many times these wounds will result in pus-filled infected areas, fever, loss of appetite, pain, and lethargy.

- Gently apply warm compresses with diluted Epsom's salts, and expel the pus from the wound by gently kneading and massaging towards the opening of the abscess.

- Keep the hole in the skin OPEN. The area beneath the skin must be allowed to drain freely.

If your pet show signs of redness, swelling, pain, loss of appetite, fever, unpleasant smell from the wound, and general lethargy, BRING YOUR PET IMMEDIATELY TO THE VETERINARIAN. Abscesses from puncture wounds can show up very quickly, in hours in some cases, and make pets very ill. Surgical drains may need to be used to achieve proper wound healing.

Holistic options:

- Massage area around visible wounds to encourage blood flow and decrease swelling.

- Arnica 30C orally for pain every six hours.

- Tarentula Cub 30C every 8 hours can from the time of the injury, in some cases, abort the formation of abscesses.

- Ledum for animal bites

- Belladonna if the wound is red, hot, and painful

- Chamomile has been traditionally used in the treatment of ruptured abscesses.

SEIZURES

Seizures occur when the brain's usual electrical activity goes awry and changes the way the body functions.

Most seizures result in the animal being on its side shaking, tremoring, or convulsing. The pet will not be aware of what it is doing and may possibly urinate or defecate during the seizure. After the main seizure, the pet will go through a period of recovery (the post-ictal period), when it is still unaware and is not responsible for its behavior.

The most important thing to do during a seizure is to keep the pet from hurting itself and to make sure you do not suffer a bite.

If a pet is close to the side of the bed or a staircase or pool, you can use pillows, blankets, or any firm surface to keep it from moving into harm's way.

Do not try to place anything near your pet's head or in its mouth. Just observe and protect your pet until the seizure AND the post-ictal period is over. Your pet will most likely recognize its name and be very tired, thirsty, scared, and disoriented when the seizure event is over.

Holistic options:

- Acupressure points for seizure and relaxation

- Aconite 30C 1 pellet every 4-8 hours

- Belladona 30C 1 pellet every 6-8 hours

Seizure

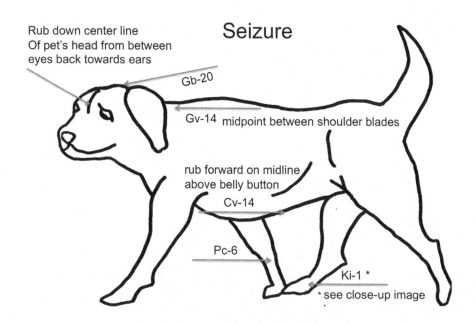

Rub down center line
Of pet's head from between
eyes back towards ears

Gb-20

Gv-14 midpoint between shoulder blades

rub forward on midline
above belly button

Cv-14

Pc-6

Ki-1 *

* see close-up image

Resuscitation Point

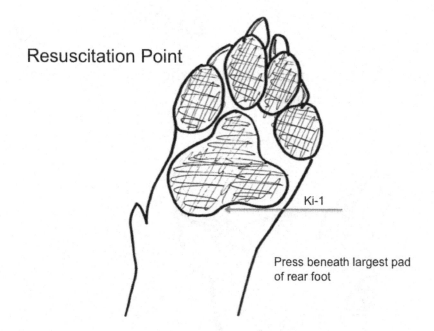

Ki-1

Press beneath largest pad
of rear foot

These points are great for relaxation and de-stressing your pet:

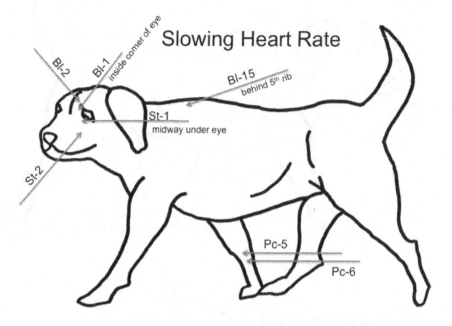

Slowing Heart Rate

Acupressure points along the top of the head also aid in relaxation:

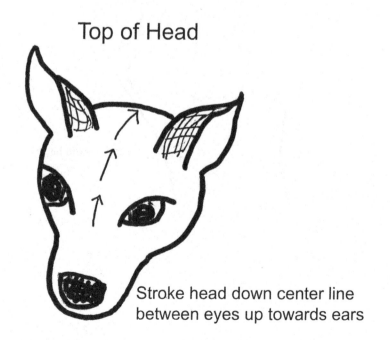

Top of Head

Stroke head down center line between eyes up towards ears

SHOCK

Shock is a life-threatening condition that may occur when blood and oxygen do not get to tissues and organs.

If you suspect shock in your pet:

1. Check gum color - The gums should be pink on most animals. Some animals have darkly-pigmented mouths, so it may be more difficult to tell. Pull up the pet's lip to check color. If the gums are pale pink or white, this is abnormal.

2. Check CRT (Capillary Refill Time) - Press on the gums gently; the pink part should turn white and then slowly come back to pink in less than 2 seconds. This is capillary refill time. If this refilling of the gum tissue takes more than 2-3 seconds or stays white, this is abnormal.

3. If the pet is slow or depressed and has cool ear tips or paws, this is abnormal.

4. Your pet may be panting.

5. Low body temperature – under 99.5°

If your pet has one or more of these signs, hold your pet so its head is slightly lower than its heart, cover with a warm towel or blanket and **rush to the emergency hospital.**

Holistic option: (to be used in conjunction with transporting to hospital)

- Place Aconitum 30c and Arnica 30c under the tongue or between the gum and the side of mouth, if it is safe to get near the mouth.

Shock

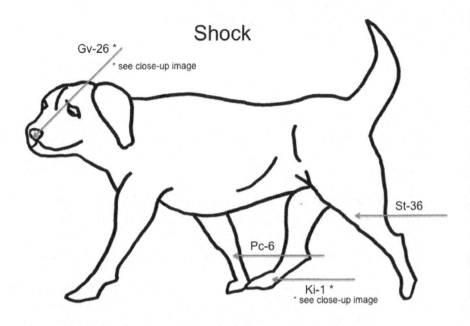

Gv-26 *
* see close-up image

St-36

Pc-6

Ki-1 *
* see close-up image

Resuscitation Point / "Hen Pecking"

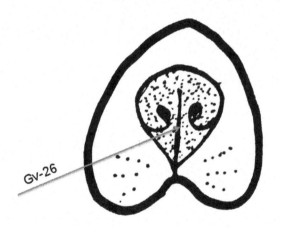

Gv-26

Resuscitation Point

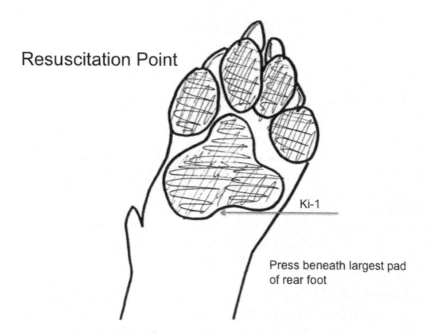

Ki-1

Press beneath largest pad
of rear foot

SLIPPED DISKS

(Aka Herniated Disk & IVDD)

Intervertebral Disk Disease (IVDD) most commonly occurs in dogs, especially in <u>chondrodystrophic</u> breeds (e.g., Dachshund, Basset Hound, Beagle, Shih Tzu, Lhasa Apso, Pekingese, and Corgi). In these dogs, there is a genetic predisposition for degeneration of the inside of the disk due to the animal's conformation, which predisposes the disk to herniation. These chondrodystrophic dogs tend to get bulging extrusions of the disk into the spinal cord.

Although most disk herniations are caused by degeneration of the disk, they can also be caused by physical trauma (an accident, such as being hit by a car). The herniation may have a very sudden onset - suddenly extruding into the spinal canal where the spinal cord runs.

In <u>non-chondrodystrophic</u> breeds, the disk degeneration starts later in life, and the herniation may occur more slowly over time (slowly protruding or bulging disk). This is commonly seen in the mid-back area, the lower-back area, and the neck area. Disk herniation in the mid-back to lower-back area may cause paralysis of the hind limbs and inability to properly urinate or defecate. Disk herniation in the neck often causes neck pain or limping on one front limb; however, it can also cause paralysis of all four limbs.

Type I and Type II Disk Disease

There are two types of disease that can afflict the intervertebral disk causing the disk to press painfully against the spinal cord.

Type I Disk Disease happens <u>quickly,</u> and as the disk material shoots upward, it presses painfully on the ligament above and potentially causes compression of the spinal cord further above.

Type II Disk Disease is a much <u>slower</u> degenerative process. Here the annulus fibrosus collapses and protrudes upward, creating a more chronic problem with pain and spinal cord compression.

Having a disk pushing against the spinal cord is an extremely painful condition, and it can happen very quickly.

Disk Disease

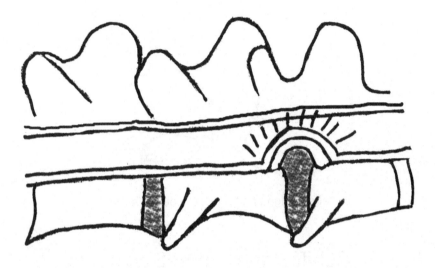

There are some very **common postures** that are seen in animals with a disk issue (Schiff Sherrington Syndrome):

- Toe dragging

- Sitting perfectly still with neck and head extended up (to relieve pressure on the spinal cord)

- Dragging the rear limbs

- Limping on one or both front limbs and having a very stiff neck

- Pain and anxiety signs such as panting, vocalization, agitation, resistance to movement.

- Schiff Sherrington Syndrome

Schiff Sherrington Syndrome
seated position

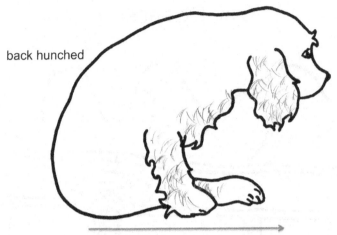

back hunched

legs straightened and extended in front

Schiff Sherrington Syndrome
standing position

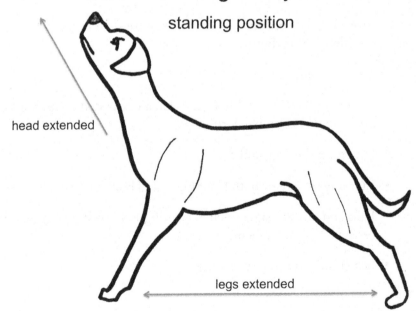

head extended

legs extended

If you notice that your pet is displaying one of these postures and seems uncomfortable, you need to **get to a veterinarian as soon as possible**. As always, safe transport for you and your pet is necessary:

If you suspect a slipped disk:

1. Keep your pet quiet and confined from extreme movements. This may avoid further spinal cord damage and pain.

2. Keep yourself safe. Your pet may bite if painful or anxious.

3. Lift the animal gently by sliding your forearm between the back legs and under the stomach, lifting your pet with the spine straight and horizontal to the ground.

4. Call a friend and arrange for transport to the hospital for evaluation. The degree of neurological damage will determine the treatment options and long-term prognosis.

Holistic options:

- Arnica Montanica 30C is very helpful for the pain of post-trauma swelling, bruising and shock.

- Ruta Graveolens 30C for muscle and ligament pain every six hours.

- Hypericum 30C to help alleviate nerve pain

Slipped Disk

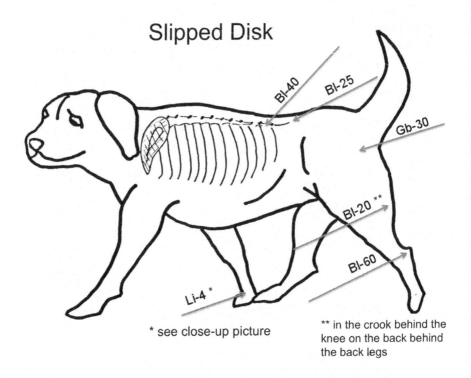

BI-40
BI-25
Gb-30
BI-20 **
BI-60
Li-4 *

* see close-up picture

** in the crook behind the knee on the back behind the back legs

Li-4

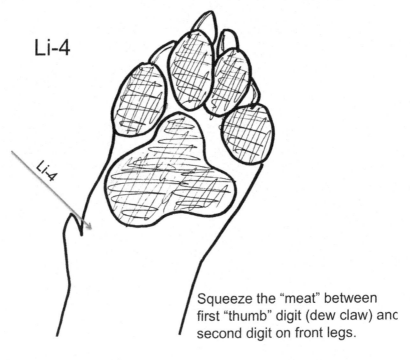

Li-4

Squeeze the "meat" between first "thumb" digit (dew claw) and second digit on front legs.

Pain

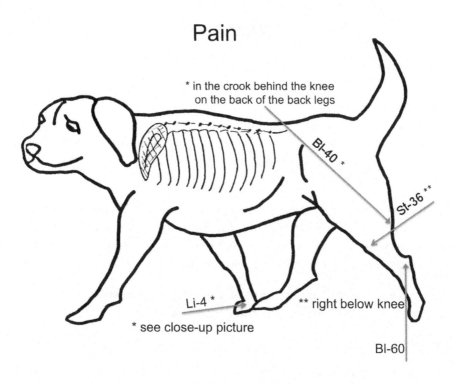

* in the crook behind the knee
on the back of the back legs

Bl-40 *

St-36 **

Li-4 *

** right below knee

* see close-up picture

Bl-60

Li-4

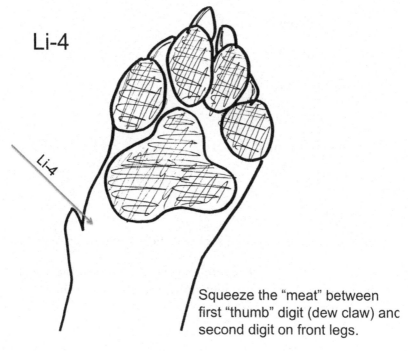

Li-4

Squeeze the "meat" between
first "thumb" digit (dew claw) anc
second digit on front legs.

SNAKEBITES

If a snake bites your pet, assume the snake is venomous, and plan to go to an emergency room. But first, restrain your pet. The shock and pain of the bite may cause your pet to lash out at itself, at surrounding people and pets, or to run.

Make every effort to keep your pet calm. This will help to slow the movement of the venom through the body. Snakebites will cause not only immediate and intense pain, but could also cause potential nerve damage and blood abnormalities, which can be fatal.

All snakebite events require **immediate veterinary assistance** to minimize the effects of the venom and control pain.

Signs of snakebites:

- Bleeding wound

- Dilated pupils

- Extreme pain

- Excitement

- Panting and drooling

- Vomiting and diarrhea

- Collapse

- Seizures

DO NOT lance the wound, suck out the wound, or use a tourniquet.

If the snake is dead, take several photos of the snake for identification at the hospital. Do not attempt this if there is any chance of injury to yourself or your pet!

Holistic options:

- Crotalus 30C – Homeopathic for rattlesnake bites – Should be given immediately after the bite event if it is safe to get into the pet without getting bitten. This homeopathic may help mitigate the effects of the bite.

- Cedron 6C for snakebites.

- Arnica 30C every eight hours.

- Echinacea (root, leaf, or flower) is traditionally used for snakebites.

⇨ **Fortunately, there are organizations that teach rattlesnake avoidance to dogs. Trainers can teach dogs to detect snakes using their senses of smell, sight, and sound and to avoid contact, which may also help dogs and owners stay out of harm's way.**

Pain

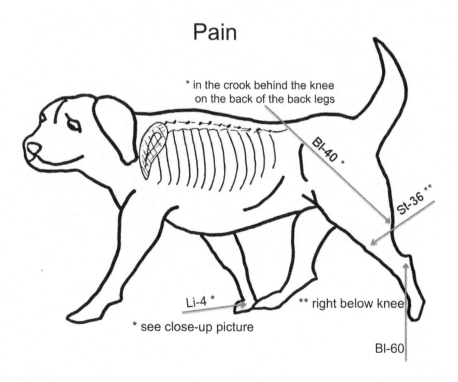

* in the crook behind the knee on the back of the back legs

Bl-40 *

St-36 **

Li-4 *

** right below knee

* see close-up picture

Bl-60

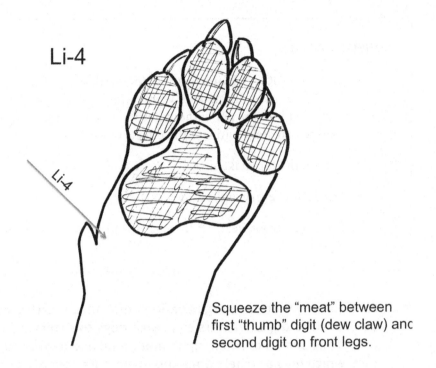

Li-4

Li-4

Squeeze the "meat" between first "thumb" digit (dew claw) and second digit on front legs.

VOMITING

Vomiting can be caused by dietary indiscretion like eating trash or poison materials. It can be cause by obstructions of the digestive tract or disorders of internal organs. Many medications and supplements can also result in vomiting, as can overexertion and heat stroke. Excessive vomiting and inability to hold down water may cause dehydration and needs to be addressed.

When food or liquids are expelled orally it is never normal. You may notice the **following indicators** prior to noticing any vomitus.

- Stomach rumbling

- Lack of energy

- "Needy" behaviors

- Eating unusual things to self-medicate (grass, plants, rocks)

- Drinking more water than usual

- Disinterest in food

- Retching

⇨ If you notice your pet retching and trying to vomit without producing any material, your pet may be experiencing a case of "Bloat" or "Gastric Dilation and Volvulus". This condition, nonproductive retching, is the number one indicator of a Bloat and is an **ABSOLUTE EMERGENCY**. Call your veterinarian or emergency hospital immediately and get prepared to transport your pet.

If you notice that your pet is vomiting, you should…

- Identify the cause.

- Rest the stomach for 12-24 hours, meaning no food.

- Stop all medications and supplements that are not absolutely necessary.

- Add electrolytes to your pet's water by adding non-flavored electrolyte drink or coconut water. Allow your pet to get small drinks of room temperature water - just enough to cover the bottom of the water bowl or an ice cube every 2 hours.

- Bismuth Subsalicylate (branded as Pepto Bismol) can be given to dogs **(NOT cats)** with vomiting or upset stomach. One teaspoon per 20 pounds every 4-6 hours.

- Check your pet's body temperature. If it is over 103°, call your veterinarian.

Many times the vomiting will remove the cause of the problem, and then the system needs to rest. <u>If vomiting lasts for more than 8-12 hours, contains blood, or your pet is weak or lethargic, seek veterinary attention.</u>

Once the vomiting subsides:

- Re-introduce food slowly, one element at a time. For example give, one protein (white meat chicken – no fat, or fish), and one carbohydrate (white or brown rice, or oatmeal). Give multiple small meals rather than any large portions.

- Give small amounts of water or teas, just enough to cover the bottom of the bowl, or make an ice cube and have your pet lick it to get the small amount of water.

- Gradually increase the portion sizes for both food and water over 24 hours until your pet can hold down food normally.

If your pet is unable to hold down food or water after 12 hours, call the veterinarian.

Holistic options:

- Peppermint and Ginger Tea can be given orally in small amounts.

- Licorice Tea helps with inflammation of the stomach

- Acupressure

- Ipecacuanha 30C – use up to three times per day for up to two days or until the clinical signs resolve.

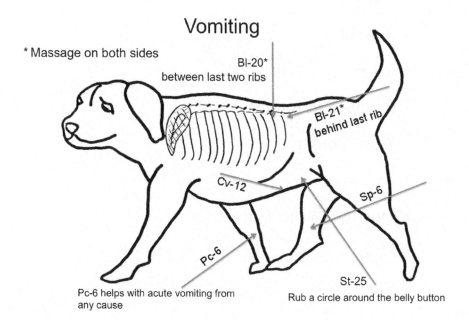

Vomiting

* Massage on both sides

Bl-20*
between last two ribs

Bl-21*
behind last rib

Cv-12

Sp-6

Pc-6

St-25

Pc-6 helps with acute vomiting from any cause

Rub a circle around the belly button

People foods your pet should never eat

Thanks to ASPCA

- Chocolate
- Coffee
- Caffeine
- Alcohol
- Avocado
- Macadamia Nuts
- Grapes and Raisins
- Yeast Dough
- Xylitol
- Onions, Garlic, Chives
- Milk
- Salt
- Nicotine
- Raw/Undercooked Meat, Eggs, and Bones

Human medications that are toxic to pets

Thanks to Pet Poison Helpline

ALWAYS call your veterinarian before you give ANY human medication to your pet!

- Pain relievers, such as Advil, Aleve, Motrin and Tylenol

- Antidepressants, such as Zoloft, Cymbalta and Effexor

- ADD / ADHD medications, such as Ritalin, Vyvanse, and Adderall

- Sleep aids, such as Klonopin, Ambien, and Lunesta

- Muscle relaxants, such as Lioresal and Flexeril

- Heart medications, such as Cartia and Cardizem

REFERENCES

Shoen, Allen M., DVM, MS. *Complementary and Alternative Veterinary Medicine.* St. Louis, MO: Mosby, Inc., 1998.

Schwartz, Cheryl DVM. *Four Paws, Five Directions.* Berkeley, CA: Celestial Arts Publishing, 1996.

Wynn, Susan G., Barbara J Fougere. *Veterinary Herbal Medicine.* St Louis, MO: Mosby Elsevier. 2007.

Wynn, Susan G.,DVM. Steve Marsden, DVM. *Manual of Natural Veterinary Medicine.* St Louis, MO: Mosby, 2003.

Sheppard, K. *The Treatment of Dogs by Homeopathy.* Essex, England: The C. W. Daniel Co. Ltd. 1972.

Heinerman, John. *Dog & Cat Care the Natural Way, Natural Pet Cures.* Paramus, NJ: Prentice Hall Press, 1998.

Null, Gary. *Natural Pet Care, How to Improve Your Animal's Quality of Life.* New York, NY: Seven Stories Press, 2000.

Fogle, Bruce. *Natural Dog Care.* New York, NY: DK Publishing, Inc. 1999.

Lane, Marion. *The Humane Society of the United States, Complete Guide to Dog Care.* Canada: Brown & Little Ltd. 1998.

Hoffman, Matthew. *Dogs: The Ultimate Care Guide.* Weldon, Inc. 1998

Hoffman, Matthew. *The Doctors Book of Home Remedies for Dogs and Cats.* Emmanus, PA: Rodale Press, Inc 1996

Roach, Peter. *The Complete Guide of Pet Care.* New York, NY: Macmillan Publishing, 1993.

Mitchell, Deborah M. DVM, MS. *"What's in your Crash Box?"* 35th International Congress of Veterinary Acupuncture, August, 2009

Marsden, Steve M, DVM, ND, MSOM, Lac, DiplCH, CVA, AHG. *Acupuncture for Feline Disorders,* International Veterinary Acupuncture Society, San Diego, CA, 2008-2009.

WaterRoverÔ by G4 Ventures www.waterrover.com

Rescue Remedy by Bach Original Flower Remedies

Mary Argo, PhD, animal communicator, www.petchat.net

Noni Lotion by Hawaiian Organic Noni, LLC

KY-Jelly by Johnson and Johnson

www.veterinarypartners.com

www.prescottpetemergency.com

www.merckmanuals.com

www.walkervalleyvet.com

CPSIA information can be obtained
at www.ICGtesting.com
Printed in the USA
FSOW03n2358290815
10458FS

9 781457 533365